INTERMITTENT FASTING FOR WOMEN OVER 50 COOKBOOK

"Elevate Your Wellness Journey with Delicious Recipes and Empowering Insights Tailored for Women Over 50"

Elizabeth J. Jaimes

Introduction

In the quiet town of Serenity Springs, lived a woman named Eleanor, a vibrant and spirited soul who had just turned 50. Eleanor had always been adventurous, and as she entered this new phase of her life, she sought ways to maintain her vitality and well-being. One day, she stumbled upon a cookbook that caught her eye – "Intermittent Fasting for Women Over 50."

Intrigued, Eleanor eagerly delved into the pages, discovering a wealth of information about the benefits of intermittent fasting tailored to her age group. The cookbook offered not just recipes but a lifestyle guide, encouraging mindful eating and embracing the changes that come with aging. Determined to embark on this new journey, Eleanor decided to give it a try.

She started her mornings with nutrient-rich smoothies from the cookbook, savoring the flavors of fresh fruits and vegetables. Eleanor found joy in preparing these meals, realizing that taking care of her body was a form of self-love.

As the days turned into weeks, Eleanor's energy levels soared. The cookbook became her trusted companion, guiding her through various fasting windows and helping her understand the importance of balanced nutrition. She explored recipes for vibrant salads and one-pan dinners, relishing the satisfaction of wholesome meals that fueled her active lifestyle.

Eleanor also discovered the community aspect of intermittent fasting. She joined online groups, sharing her experiences and learning from others. The cookbook had not only become a source of delicious recipes but a catalyst for connection and support.

Her newfound routine wasn't just about the physical changes; Eleanor embraced mindfulness in her eating habits. The cookbook emphasized the significance of enjoying meals with gratitude and savoring every bite. This holistic approach transformed Eleanor's relationship with food, bringing a sense of fulfillment and joy to her daily life.

With each passing month, Eleanor felt a renewed sense of vitality. Her friends noticed the positive changes and marveled at her radiant spirit. She became an advocate for healthy living, sharing the cookbook with those around her.

Eleanor's journey with intermittent fasting became more than just a health choice; it became a celebration of life and the wisdom that comes with age. As she continued to savor the flavors of her newfound lifestyle, Eleanor discovered that age was just a number, and the pages of the cookbook held the recipe for a fulfilling and vibrant life.

Welcome to the "Intermittent Fasting for Women Over 50 Cookbook," a guide crafted with care to empower and inspire women on a journey toward vibrant health and well-being. This cookbook is not just a collection of recipes; it's a companion on your path to embracing the benefits of intermittent fasting tailored to the unique needs of women over 50.
As we navigate the intricacies of life's different chapters, our approach to health and nutrition evolves. This cookbook is designed to celebrate the wisdom and vitality that come with age, offering a holistic perspective on intermittent fasting that goes beyond mere dietary choices. It's a roadmap for nourishing your body, mind, and spirit.

Within these pages, you'll find a carefully curated selection of recipes that are not only delicious but also thoughtfully designed to meet the nutritional requirements of women in this phase of life. From nutrient-rich smoothies to balanced one-pan dinners, each dish is a celebration of flavor and well-being.

But this cookbook is more than just a culinary guide. It's an invitation to embrace a lifestyle that encompasses mindful eating, fostering a deeper connection with your body and the nourishment it deserves. Discover the joy of savoring each bite, and let this cookbook be a source of inspiration as you embark on a journey toward a healthier and more fulfilling life.

Whether you're new to intermittent fasting or seeking to enhance your existing practices, this cookbook is here to support you. Let it be a source of encouragement, a companion in your kitchen, and a testament to the vitality that can be found at any age. Welcome to a world where food is not just sustenance but a celebration of life's abundance.

Overview of Intermittent Fasting

Intermittent fasting is an eating pattern that cycles between periods of eating and fasting. Unlike traditional diets that focus on what you eat, intermittent fasting emphasizes when you eat. This approach doesn't prescribe specific foods but rather dictates when to consume them.

The primary goal of intermittent fasting is to optimize the body's metabolic processes, promote cellular repair, and enhance overall health. It has gained popularity for its potential benefits, including weight management, improved insulin sensitivity, and longevity.

There are various methods of intermittent fasting, each involving specific time frames for eating and fasting. Common approaches include the 16/8 method, where you fast for 16 hours and have an 8-hour eating window, and the 5:2 method, which involves eating regularly for five days and significantly reducing caloric intake for two non-consecutive days.

Research suggests that intermittent fasting may positively impact various aspects of health, such as cardiovascular function, brain health, and inflammation reduction. It is essential to note that individual responses may vary, and consulting with a healthcare professional before starting any fasting regimen is advised, especially for specific populations, such as women over 50.

This overview serves as a starting point to explore the world of intermittent fasting, providing insights into its principles, potential benefits, and considerations for implementation. As you delve into this approach, remember to prioritize balance, nourishment, and mindfulness in your journey toward improved well-being.

Benefits for Women Over 50

Intermittent fasting can offer a range of potential benefits for women in the dynamic phase of life beyond 50. While individual responses may vary, here are some advantages that women may experience:

1. **Weight Management**: Intermittent fasting may assist in weight regulation by promoting fat loss while preserving lean muscle mass. This can be particularly beneficial for maintaining a healthy body composition.

2. **Improved Metabolic Health**: Fasting periods may enhance insulin sensitivity, potentially reducing the risk of insulin resistance and Type 2 diabetes. This can be crucial for managing metabolic health, especially as women age.
3. **Enhanced Cognitive Function**: Some studies suggest that intermittent fasting may support brain health by promoting the production of brain-derived neurotrophic factor (BDNF), a protein associated with cognitive function and the growth of new neurons.

4. **Heart Health**: Intermittent fasting may contribute to cardiovascular health by improving lipid profiles, reducing blood pressure, and supporting overall heart function.

5. **Hormonal Balance**: Fasting periods might influence hormonal balance, which is particularly relevant for women going through hormonal changes post-menopause. It may contribute to the regulation of hormones such as insulin and growth hormone.

6. **Inflammation Reduction**: Intermittent fasting has been linked to a reduction in inflammation markers. Chronic inflammation is associated with various age-related conditions, and mitigating it can be crucial for overall health.

7. **Cellular Repair**: Fasting triggers autophagy, a cellular process that involves the removal of damaged cells and cellular components. This renewal process may contribute to longevity and the prevention of age-related diseases.

8. **Longevity**: While research is ongoing, some studies suggest that intermittent fasting may be linked to increased lifespan and improved longevity.

Understanding Your Nutritional Needs

As women transition beyond the age of 50, a thoughtful consideration of nutritional needs becomes increasingly vital. Recognizing and addressing these needs can significantly impact overall health and well-being. Here are key factors to consider:

1. **Caloric Requirements**: Metabolic changes associated with aging may affect caloric needs. Understanding your individual energy requirements based on factors like activity level, metabolism, and muscle mass is essential for maintaining a healthy weight.

2. **Protein Intake**: Adequate protein is crucial for preserving muscle mass, supporting immune function, and promoting satiety. Women over 50 should focus on incorporating lean protein sources into their diets, such as poultry, fish, beans, and dairy.

3. **Calcium and Vitamin D:** Bone health becomes a priority with age, making sufficient calcium and vitamin D intake essential. Dairy products, leafy greens, and fortified foods are excellent sources to support bone density.

4. **Fiber-Rich Foods**: Maintaining digestive health becomes increasingly important. Including fiber-rich

foods like whole grains, fruits, and vegetables aids in digestion, supports gut health, and may contribute to weight management.

5. **Hydration**: Staying adequately hydrated is crucial for overall health. Women over 50 should pay attention to their fluid intake, incorporating water-rich foods and beverages throughout the day.

6. **Healthy Fats**: Focus on incorporating sources of healthy fats, such as avocados, nuts, and olive oil. These fats are essential for hormone production and absorption of fat-soluble vitamins.

7. **Micronutrients**: Ensure a diverse and colorful array of fruits and vegetables to obtain a broad spectrum of essential vitamins and minerals. These nutrients play key roles in various bodily functions and contribute to overall well-being.

8. **Adapt to Dietary Preferences and Restrictions:** Consider any dietary preferences, intolerances, or restrictions you may have. Tailoring your nutritional approach to accommodate these factors ensures a sustainable and enjoyable dietary pattern.

Choosing the Right Intermittent Fasting Plan

Embarking on an intermittent fasting journey involves selecting a plan that aligns with your lifestyle, preferences, and health goals. Here's a guide to help you navigate the various intermittent fasting methods:

1. **16/8 Method (Time-Restricted Eating):**
   How it works: Fasting for 16 hours daily and restricting your eating to an 8-hour window.
   Suitability: Well-suited for beginners and those looking for a straightforward approach. Ideal for individuals who prefer a consistent daily routine.

2. **5:2 Diet (Modified Fasting):**
   How it works: Eating normally for five days and consuming a reduced calorie intake (around 500-600 calories) on two non-consecutive days.
   Suitability: Suitable for those who prefer periodic fasting. It provides flexibility but requires planning on fasting days.

3. **Eat-Stop-Eat**:
   How it works: Involves a 24-hour fast once or twice a week, with no calorie intake during the fasting period.

Suitability: Suited for individuals comfortable with longer fasting periods. May require adaptation for those new to fasting.

4. **Alternate-Day Fasting:**

How it works: Alternating between days of regular eating and days of either full or modified fasting.

Suitability: Suitable for those who appreciate variety in their fasting routine but may pose a challenge for sustained adherence.

5. **Warrior Diet:**

How it works: Involves eating small amounts of raw fruits and vegetables during the day and consuming one large meal at night within a 4-hour eating window.

Suitability: Suited for those who prefer one substantial evening meal. It requires discipline during the daytime fasting period.

6. **OMAD (One Meal a Day):**

How it works: Restricting all food intake to a single meal within a 1-hour window each day.

Suitability: Suited for those comfortable with prolonged daily fasting. It requires careful meal planning to ensure nutritional needs are met.

Preparing Your Kitchen for Intermittent Fasting Success

Creating a supportive environment in your kitchen is a key step toward a successful intermittent fasting journey. Here's a guide to help you prepare your kitchen for a seamless and enjoyable experience:

1. **Stock Up on Essential Ingredients**:
   - Ensure your pantry is well-stocked with nutritious, non-perishable items like whole grains, legumes, nuts, and seeds.
   - Fill your refrigerator with fresh produce, lean proteins, and dairy or plant-based alternatives.

2. **Invest in Quality Kitchen Tools:**
   - Equip your kitchen with tools that simplify meal preparation, such as a sharp knife, cutting board, blender for smoothies, and non-stick cookware.
   - Consider a kitchen scale for portion control and accurate ingredient measurements.

3. **Organize Your Fridge and Pantry:**
   - Arrange your kitchen spaces to make healthier choices more accessible. Place fresh produce at eye level in the fridge and keep snacks like nuts readily available.

- Label and organize containers to store prepped ingredients, making it easier to assemble meals during eating windows.

4. **Meal Prep for Convenience:**

- Dedicate time each week to meal prepping. Cook and portion meals ahead of time to have healthy options readily available.
- Prepare grab-and-go snacks, such as cut vegetables or pre-portioned nuts, for quick and convenient choices during eating windows.

5. **Experiment with Intermittent Fasting Recipes**:

- Explore recipes that align with your chosen intermittent fasting plan. Look for meals that are nutrient-dense and satisfying to support your nutritional needs.
- Keep a collection of go-to recipes that make meal planning enjoyable.

6. **Stay Hydrated:**

- Ensure your kitchen is stocked with plenty of water. Consider infusing water with herbs or fruits to add a refreshing twist.
- Herbal teas can be excellent additions during fasting periods to stay hydrated without consuming calories.

7. **Mindful Eating Environment**:
   - Create a pleasant and mindful eating space. Eliminate distractions during meals to focus on savoring your food.
   - Consider incorporating soft lighting and calming elements to enhance the dining experience.

8. **Educate Yourself on Labels:**
   - Familiarize yourself with food labels to make informed choices. Pay attention to portion sizes, nutritional content, and ingredients.

Essential Ingredients for Intermittent Fasting Success

Stocking your kitchen with nutrient-dense and versatile ingredients is crucial for a successful intermittent fasting journey. Here's a list of essential ingredients to keep on hand:

1. **Whole Grains:**
   - Quinoa
   - Brown rice
   - Oats
   - Barley

2. **Lean Proteins**:
   - Chicken breast
   - Turkey
   - Fish (salmon, tuna)
   - Lean cuts of beef or pork
   - Plant-based proteins (tofu, tempeh, legumes)

3. **Healthy Fats:**
   - Avocado
   - Olive oil
   - Nuts (almonds, walnuts)
   - Seeds (chia seeds, flaxseeds)

4. **Fresh Produce**:

- Leafy greens (spinach, kale, arugula)
- Colorful vegetables (bell peppers, broccoli, carrots)
- Fresh fruits (berries, apples, citrus)

5. Dairy or Dairy Alternatives:
- Greek yogurt
- Cottage cheese
- Almond or coconut milk

6. Herbs and Spices:
- Fresh herbs (basil, cilantro, mint)
- Spices (turmeric, cumin, paprika)
- Garlic and ginger

7. Eggs:
- A versatile protein source for various dishes.

8. Low-Calorie Sweeteners:
- Stevia or monk fruit for sweetening without added calories.

9. Whole-Grain Products:
- Whole-grain bread
- Whole-grain pasta
- Quinoa or whole-grain wraps

10. **Hydration Options:**
   - Water
   - Herbal teas
   - Sparkling water

11. **Canned Goods:**
   - Canned beans (black beans, chickpeas)
   - Canned tomatoes
   - Low-sodium broths

12. **Condiments and Sauces:**
   - Mustard
   - Hot sauce
   - Olive tapenade
   - Low-sodium soy sauce or tamari

13. **Sweeteners:**
   - Honey or maple syrup (use in moderation)
   - Vanilla extract

14. **Frozen Vegetables and Fruits:**
   - Convenient for quick and easy meal preparation.

15. **Nutritional Extras:**
   - Nutritional yeast (for a savory, cheese-like flavor)
   - Apple cider vinegar
   - Dark chocolate (70% cocoa or higher)

Kitchen Tools for Intermittent Fasting Success

Equipping your kitchen with the right tools can make meal preparation and intermittent fasting more enjoyable and efficient. Here's a list of essential kitchen tools to support your journey:

1. **Quality Blender:**
   - Ideal for preparing nutrient-packed smoothies and shakes.

2. **Sharp Knives and Cutting Board:**
   - Essential for safe and efficient chopping, slicing, and dicing.

3. **Non-Stick Cookware:**
   - Make cooking and cleaning a breeze while minimizing the need for excessive oils.

4. **Food Scale:**
   - Helpful for portion control and accurate measurement of ingredients.

5. **Measuring Cups and Spoons:**
   - Ensure precise quantities for cooking and baking.
6. **Steamer Basket:**

- Perfect for retaining nutrients in vegetables while keeping them crisp.

7. Food Processor:
   - Useful for chopping, blending, and preparing various ingredients.

8. High-Quality Pots and Pans:
   - Invest in durable cookware for even cooking and longevity.

9. Slow Cooker:
   - Convenient for preparing flavorful meals with minimal effort.

10. Salad Spinner:
   - Ensures dry and crisp greens for refreshing salads.

11. Instant-Read Thermometer:
   - Useful for checking the doneness of proteins.

12. Spiralizer:
   - Create vegetable noodles for healthier alternatives to pasta.

13. Citrus Juicer:
   - Extract fresh juice for recipes and beverages.

14. **Baking Sheets and Pans:**
   - Essential for roasting vegetables or preparing baked dishes.

15. **Grill Pan:**
   - Mimic the flavor of outdoor grilling indoors.

16. **Air Fryer:**
   - Cook with less oil for crispy and healthier results.

17. **Kitchen Timer:**
   - Helps you stay on track with fasting and eating windows.

18. **Mason Jars and Containers**:
   - Perfect for storing prepped ingredients and meals.

19. **Silicone Baking Mats:**
   - Provide a non-stick surface for baking without added oils.

20. **Vegetable Peeler:**
   - Easily peel and prepare a variety of vegetables.

21. **Strainer/Colander**:
   - Essential for draining pasta, washing produce, and more.

22. **Tongs and Spatulas:**
   - Versatile tools for flipping and turning ingredients.

23. **Kitchen Utensil Set:**
   - Includes spoons, ladles, and spatulas for various cooking needs.

24. **Wine Opener:**
   - For those occasional moments of indulgence.

Nourishing Breakfast Recipes for Intermittent Fasting

Start your day with energy and flavor by trying these wholesome and satisfying breakfast recipes tailored for intermittent fasting:

1. **Protein-Packed Smoothie Bowl:**
   Ingredients:
     - 1 cup unsweetened almond milk
     - 1 scoop protein powder
     - 1 frozen banana
     - Handful of berries
     - Toppings: granola, chia seeds, sliced almonds

2. **Avocado and Egg Breakfast Wrap:**
   Ingredients:
     - Whole-grain wrap
     - 1/2 avocado, mashed
     - 1 boiled egg, sliced
     - Fresh spinach leaves
     - Salsa for added flavor

3. **Greek Yogurt Parfait:**
   Ingredients:
     - 1 cup Greek yogurt
     - Fresh berries (blueberries, strawberries)

- Granola for crunch
- Drizzle of honey

4. Quinoa Breakfast Bowl:
Ingredients:
- Cooked quinoa
- Sliced banana
- Chopped nuts (walnuts or almonds)
- Dash of cinnamon
- Splash of almond milk

5. Smoked Salmon and Avocado Toast:
Ingredients:
- Whole-grain toast
- Smoked salmon
- Sliced avocado
- Fresh dill and a squeeze of lemon

6. Chia Seed Pudding:
Ingredients:
- 2 tbsp chia seeds
- 1 cup unsweetened almond milk
- Fresh berries
- Optional: a drizzle of maple syrup

7. Vegetable Omelette:
-Ingredients:
- 2 eggs
- Mixed vegetables (bell peppers, spinach, tomatoes)

- Feta or goat cheese
- Fresh herbs (parsley or chives)

8. **Whole-Grain Pancakes:**
   Ingredients:
   - Whole-grain pancake mix
   - Sliced bananas
   - Chopped nuts (pecans or almonds)
   - Greek yogurt topping

Nutrient-Rich Smoothie Recipes for a Boost of Energy

Elevate your mornings with these nutrient-packed smoothie recipes designed to fuel your body and kickstart your day during intermittent fasting:

1. **Green Goddess Smoothie:**
   Ingredients:
     - Handful of spinach
     - 1/2 cucumber, peeled
     - 1 green apple, cored
     - 1/2 lemon, juiced
     - 1 cup coconut water
     - Ice cubes

2. **Berry Bliss Smoothie:**
   Ingredients:
     - Mixed berries (strawberries, blueberries, raspberries)
     - 1/2 banana
     - 1 cup almond milk
     - 1 tablespoon chia seeds
     - Greek yogurt for creaminess

3. **Tropical Paradise Smoothie:**
   Ingredients:
     - Pineapple chunks

- Mango slices
- Coconut water or coconut milk
- 1/2 lime, juiced
- Handful of kale

4. **Protein-Packed Peanut Butter Smoothie:**
   Ingredients:
   - 1 scoop protein powder (vanilla or chocolate)
   - 2 tablespoons peanut butter
   - 1 banana
   - 1 cup almond milk
   - Ice cubes

5. ***Citrus Sunrise Smoothie:**
   Ingredients:
   - Orange segments
   - 1/2 grapefruit, peeled
   - 1 carrot, chopped
   - 1/2 inch ginger, grated
   - Water or orange juice

6. **Chocolate Banana Almond Smoothie**:
   Ingredients:
   - 1 banana

- 1 tablespoon almond butter
- 1 tablespoon cacao powder
- 1 cup unsweetened almond milk
- Ice cubes

7. **Antioxidant-Rich Acai Berry Smoothie:**
   Ingredients:
   - Acai berry puree (frozen or unsweetened)
   - Mixed berries
   - 1 tablespoon hemp seeds
   - Coconut water or almond milk

8. **Vanilla Coffee Protein Smoothie:**
   Ingredients:
   - 1 cup brewed and cooled coffee
   - 1 scoop vanilla protein powder
   - 1 tablespoon almond butter
   - Ice cubes

Energizing Breakfast Bowl Ideas for Intermittent Fasting

Fuel your mornings with these energizing and nutritious breakfast bowl recipes, perfectly suited for intermittent fasting:

1. **Power-Packed Acai Bowl:**
   Ingredients:
     - Acai berry puree (frozen or unsweetened)
     - Banana slices
     - Granola
     - Chia seeds
     - Coconut flakes
     - Almond butter drizzle

2. **Greek Yogurt and Fruit Bowl:**
   Ingredients:
     - Greek yogurt
     - Mixed berries (strawberries, blueberries,
raspberries)
     - Honey drizzle
     - Almonds or walnuts
     - Granola for crunch

3. **Savory Breakfast Quinoa Bowl:**
   Ingredients:
     - Cooked quinoa
     - Sautéed spinach and cherry tomatoes
     - Poached egg
     - Avocado slices
     - Feta cheese crumbles

4. **Smoothie Bowl with Toppings:**
   Ingredients:
   - Your favorite smoothie base
   - Sliced kiwi, banana, and berries
   - Granola
   - Chia seeds
   - Shredded coconut

5. **Chia Seed Pudding Bowl:**
   Ingredients:
   - Chia seed pudding (made with almond milk)
   - Mango chunks
   - Kiwi slices
   - Pistachios or almonds
   - Coconut flakes

6. **Warm Oatmeal Bowl with Nut Butter:**
   Ingredients:
   - Steel-cut oats
   - Almond or peanut butter
   - Sliced banana
   - Cinnamon sprinkle
   - Hemp seeds

7. **Mexican-Inspired Breakfast Bowl:**
   Ingredients:

- Scrambled eggs with diced peppers and onions
- Black beans
- Avocado slices
- Salsa
- Cilantro garnish

8. **Mango Coconut Rice Pudding Bowl:**
   Ingredients:
   - Coconut milk rice pudding
   - Fresh mango chunks
   - Toasted coconut flakes
   - Cashews or macadamia nuts

Nutrient-Packed Lunch Ideas for Intermittent Fasting

Enjoy these satisfying and nutritious lunch ideas that align with intermittent fasting principles:

1. **Grilled Chicken Salad:**
   - Grilled chicken breast
   - Mixed greens (spinach, arugula, romaine)
   - Cherry tomatoes
   - Cucumber slices
   - Avocado
   - Balsamic vinaigrette dressing

2. **Quinoa and Chickpea Bowl:**
   - Cooked quinoa
   - Chickpeas (roasted for extra crunch)
   - Roasted vegetables (zucchini, bell peppers, cherry tomatoes)
   - Feta cheese
   - Lemon-tahini dressing

3. **Vegetarian Wrap:**
   - Whole-grain wrap
   - Hummus spread
   - Sliced cucumber, bell peppers, and tomatoes
   - Feta cheese
   - Kalamata olives

4. **Salmon and Avocado Wrap:**
   - Grilled or baked salmon
   - Whole-grain wrap
   - Avocado slices
   - Mixed greens
   - Greek yogurt dill sauce

5. **Mediterranean Quinoa Salad:**
   - Quinoa
   - Cherry tomatoes
   - Cucumber
   - Red onion
   - Kalamata olives
   - Feta cheese

- Olive oil and lemon dressing

6. **Turkey and Veggie Lettuce Wraps:**
   - Ground turkey sautéed with onions and garlic
   - Lettuce leaves as wraps
   - Shredded carrots
   - Sliced bell peppers
   - Hoisin sauce drizzle

7. **Chickpea and Spinach Stew:**
   - Chickpeas
   - Sautéed spinach
   - Diced tomatoes
   - Garlic and onion
   - Vegetable broth
   - Cumin and paprika for seasoning

8. **Sweet Potato and Black Bean Bowl:**
   - Roasted sweet potato cubes
   - Black beans
   - Corn kernels
   - Avocado slices
   - Lime-cilantro dressing

Healthy Salad Ideas for Intermittent Fasting

Savor the freshness with these nutrient-rich and delicious salad ideas that make for satisfying meals during intermittent fasting:

1. **Summer Berry Spinach Salad:**
   - Baby spinach
   - Mixed berries (strawberries, blueberries, raspberries)
   - Goat cheese crumbles
   - Candied walnuts or almonds
   - Balsamic vinaigrette dressing

2. **Mango Avocado Quinoa Salad:**
   - Cooked quinoa
   - Mango chunks
   - Avocado slices
   - Red onion, thinly sliced
   - Cilantro
   - Lime vinaigrette dressing

3. **Caprese Salad with a Twist:**
   - Fresh mozzarella balls
   - Cherry tomatoes
   - Basil leaves
   - Avocado slices
   - Balsamic glaze drizzle

4. **Kale and Roasted Vegetable Salad:**
   - Massaged kale leaves
   - Roasted sweet potatoes, carrots, and Brussels
sprouts
   - Pomegranate seeds
   - Feta cheese
   - Lemon-tahini dressing

5. **Greek Salad with Quinoa:**
   - Quinoa
   - Cherry tomatoes
   - Cucumber
   - Kalamata olives
   - Red onion
   - Feta cheese
   - Greek dressing

6. **Tuna and White Bean Salad:**
   - Canned tuna, drained
   - White beans (cannellini or navy)
   - Cherry tomatoes
   - Red onion
   - Fresh parsley
   - Lemon-olive oil dressing

7. **Asian-Inspired Chicken Salad:**
   - Grilled chicken breast

- Mixed greens
- Shredded cabbage and carrots
- Edamame
- Sesame seeds
- Ginger-soy dressing

8. **Roasted Beet and Goat Cheese Salad:**
   - Roasted beets, sliced
   - Mixed greens
   - Walnuts or pecans
   - Goat cheese crumbles
   - Balsamic vinaigrette dressing

Protein-Packed Wrap Ideas for Satisfying Meals

Wrap up your nutrition with these protein-rich and flavorful wrap ideas, perfect for keeping you fueled during your eating window in intermittent fasting:

1. **Chicken Caesar Wrap:**
   - Grilled chicken strips

- Romaine lettuce
- Parmesan cheese
- Whole-grain wrap
- Caesar dressing

2. **Vegetarian Hummus Wrap:**
   - Hummus spread
   - Sliced cucumber
   - Cherry tomatoes
   - Red onion
   - Feta cheese
   - Whole-grain or spinach wrap

3. **Turkey and Avocado Wrap**:
   - Sliced turkey breast
   - Avocado slices
   - Spinach leaves
   - Tomato slices
   - Whole-grain wrap
   - Dijon mustard or Greek yogurt sauce

4. **BLT Wrap with Turkey**:
   - Turkey bacon
   - Lettuce
   - Tomato slices
   - Grilled chicken or turkey slices
   - Whole-grain wrap
   - Light mayo or avocado spread

5. **Mediterranean Chickpea Wrap:**
   - Chickpea salad (mashed chickpeas, cucumber, cherry tomatoes, red onion, olives)
   - Feta cheese
   - Spinach leaves
   - Whole-grain wrap
   - Tzatziki sauce

6. **Salmon and Avocado Wrap:**
   - Grilled or baked salmon
   - Avocado slices
   - Mixed greens
   - Whole-grain wrap
   - Lemon-dill yogurt sauce

7. **Egg Salad Spinach Wrap:**
   - Egg salad (hard-boiled eggs, Greek yogurt, mustard)
   - Spinach leaves
   - Whole-grain wrap
   - Sprouts for added crunch

8. **BBQ Chicken Wrap:**
   - Shredded BBQ chicken
   - Coleslaw mix (cabbage and carrots)

- Whole-grain wrap
- BBQ sauce drizzle

Delicious Dinner Ideas for Intermittent Fasting

Wrap up your day with these flavorful and satisfying dinner ideas that align with intermittent fasting principles:

1. **Grilled Salmon with Quinoa and Asparagus:**
   - Grilled salmon fillet
   - Quinoa
   - Roasted asparagus
   - Lemon-dill sauce

2. **Vegetarian Stir-Fry with Tofu:**
   - Stir-fried tofu
   - Assorted colorful vegetables (broccoli, bell peppers, snap peas)
   - Brown rice or cauliflower rice
   - Soy-ginger sauce

3. **Mushroom and Spinach Stuffed Chicken Breast:**
   - Chicken breast stuffed with sautéed mushrooms and spinach

- Roasted sweet potatoes
- Steamed green beans

4. Spaghetti Squash with Turkey Bolognese:
- Roasted spaghetti squash strands
- Lean ground turkey Bolognese sauce
- Fresh basil and grated Parmesan

5. Baked Cod with Quinoa Salad:
- Baked cod fillet
- Quinoa salad with cherry tomatoes, cucumber, and feta
- Lemon-tahini dressing

6. Chickpea and Vegetable Curry:
- Chickpea and vegetable curry
- Quinoa or brown rice
- Fresh cilantro for garnish

7. Shrimp and Avocado Salad:
- Grilled shrimp
- Avocado slices
- Mixed greens
- Cherry tomatoes
- Cilantro-lime vinaigrette

8. Beef and Broccoli Stir-Fry:
- Stir-fried beef strips

- Broccoli florets
- Brown rice or cauliflower rice
- Teriyaki or soy-ginger sauce

Healthy Snacks and Sweets for Intermittent Fasting

Satisfy your cravings with these nutritious snack and sweet ideas that fit well into your intermittent fasting routine:

Snack Ideas:

1. **Greek Yogurt Parfait:**
   - Greek yogurt
   - Fresh berries
   - Granola
   - Drizzle of honey

2. **Sliced Apple with Almond Butter**:
   - Apple slices
   - Almond or peanut butter

3. **Hard-Boiled Eggs:**
   - Protein-packed and convenient.

4. **Mixed Nuts:**

- Almonds, walnuts, pistachios, or a mix.

5. Hummus and Veggie Sticks:
   - Carrot, cucumber, and bell pepper sticks with hummus.

6. Cheese and Whole-Grain Crackers:
   - Pair low-fat cheese with whole-grain crackers.

7. Protein Smoothie:
   - Blend protein powder, almond milk, and a handful of berries.

8. Cottage Cheese with Pineapple:
   - Cottage cheese with fresh pineapple chunks.

Sweet Treats:

1. Dark Chocolate and Berries:
   - Dark chocolate squares with a side of fresh berries.

2. Chia Seed Pudding with Fruit:
   - Chia seed pudding topped with sliced strawberries or mango.

3. Banana Ice Cream:
   - Frozen banana blended into a creamy, ice cream-like consistency.

4. **Yogurt-Dipped Strawberries:**
   - Dip strawberries in Greek yogurt and freeze.

5. **Baked Cinnamon Apple Slices:**
   - Thin apple slices baked with cinnamon.

6. **Trail Mix:**
   - A mix of nuts, seeds, and dried fruits.

7. **Energy Balls:**
   - Combine dates, nuts, and cocoa powder into bite-sized energy balls.

8. **Berries with Whipped Coconut Cream**:
   - Fresh berries served with a dollop of whipped coconut cream.

Nourishing Snack Ideas for Intermittent Fasting

Keep your energy levels up with these nourishing and satisfying snack ideas tailored for intermittent fasting:

1. ***Avocado Toast on Whole-Grain Crackers:**
   - Mashed avocado on whole-grain crackers.
   - Optional toppings: cherry tomatoes, radish slices, or a sprinkle of sea salt.

2. **Cucumber and Hummus Bites:**
   - Cucumber slices with a dollop of hummus.
   - Top with a sprinkle of paprika or fresh herbs.

3. **Trail Mix with a Twist:**
   - Mix almonds, walnuts, pumpkin seeds, and dried berries.
   - Add a touch of dark chocolate for a sweet element.

4. **Greek Yogurt with Berries and Nuts:**
   - Greek yogurt topped with fresh berries and a handful of mixed nuts.
   - Drizzle with honey for sweetness.

5. **Edamame Snack:**
   - Steamed edamame pods sprinkled with sea salt.
   - A great source of plant-based protein.

6. **Apple Nachos:**
   - Apple slices arranged on a plate.
   - Drizzle with almond butter and sprinkle with granola.

7. **Rice Cake with Nut Butter and Banana:**
   - Brown rice cake spread with almond or peanut butter.
   - Top with banana slices.

8. **Caprese Skewers:**

- Cherry tomatoes, mozzarella balls, and fresh basil leaves on toothpicks.
   - Drizzle with balsamic glaze.

9. **Roasted Chickpeas:**
   - Roast chickpeas with olive oil and your favorite spices.
   - A crunchy and satisfying snack.

10. **Carrot Sticks with Guacamole:**
   - Fresh carrot sticks paired with homemade guacamole.
   - Guacamole can include diced tomatoes, onions, and lime juice.

Guilt-Free Dessert Ideas for Intermittent Fasting

Indulge in these satisfying and healthier dessert options that won't derail your intermittent fasting efforts:

1. **Chocolate-Dipped Strawberries:**
   - Dip fresh strawberries in dark chocolate.
   - Enjoy in moderation for a sweet treat.

2. **Frozen Banana Bites:**
   - Slice bananas and dip in yogurt.

   - Freeze for a creamy, bite-sized dessert.

3. Chia Seed Pudding Parfait:
   - Layer chia seed pudding with fresh fruit and a sprinkle of granola.

4. Greek Yogurt Berry Bark:
   - Mix Greek yogurt with berries and spread on a baking sheet.
   - Freeze and break into pieces for a yogurt bark.

5. Baked Cinnamon Apples:
   - Slice apples and bake with cinnamon until tender.
   - Top with a dollop of Greek yogurt.

6. Date and Nut Energy Balls:
   - Blend dates, nuts, and a touch of cocoa powder.
   - Roll into bite-sized energy balls.

7. Coconut Bliss Balls:
   - Combine shredded coconut, almond flour, and a sweetener.
   - Form into small balls and refrigerate.

8. Fruit Sorbet:
   - Blend frozen fruits like berries or mango.
   - Serve as a refreshing sorbet.

9. **Protein Ice Cream:**
   - Mix protein powder with almond milk and freeze.
   - Scoop for a protein-packed ice cream alternative.

10. **Avocado Chocolate Mousse:**
   - Blend avocado, cocoa powder, and a sweetener.
   - Chill for a creamy chocolate mousse.

Effective Fasting Strategies for Intermittent Fasting

Intermittent fasting involves cycling between periods of eating and fasting. Here are popular fasting strategies to consider:

1. **16/8 Method (Leangains Protocol):**
   - Fast for 16 hours daily and have an 8-hour eating window.
   - Example: Eat between 12:00 pm and 8:00 pm, then fast until the next day at 12:00 pm.

2. **5:2 Diet:**
   - Eat normally for five days a week.
   - Limit caloric intake to around 500-600 calories on two non-consecutive fasting days.

3. **Alternate-Day Fasting:**
   - Alternate between days of regular eating and days of significant calorie reduction or complete fasting.

4. **Eat-Stop-Eat**:
   - Implement a 24-hour fast once or twice a week.
   - Example: Eat dinner at 7:00 pm and then refrain from eating until the next day's dinner at 7:00 pm.

5. **Warrior Diet:**
   - Eat small amounts of raw fruits and vegetables during the day.
   - Consume one large meal at night within a 4-hour eating window.

6. **OMAD (One Meal a Day):**
   - Consume all daily calories in a single meal, usually within a one-hour eating window.
   - This approach often involves a 23:1 fasting-to-eating ratio.

7. **Spontaneous Meal Skipping:**
   - Skip meals when not hungry or when it fits your schedule.
   - Allows for flexibility without rigid fasting windows.

8. **Extended Fasting (48 hours or more):**
   - Occasionally extend the fasting period to 48 hours or more for enhanced autophagy and metabolic benefits.

Tips for Successful Intermittent Fasting

1. **Stay Hydrated:**
   - **Drink plenty of** water during fasting periods to stay hydrated and help control hunger.

2. **Choose Nutrient-Dense Foods:**
   - Opt for whole, nutrient-dense foods during eating windows to support overall health.

3. **Gradual Adaptation:**
   - If new to fasting, start with shorter fasting periods and gradually increase as your body adjusts.

4. **Listen to Your Body:**
   - Pay attention to hunger and fullness cues. Eat when hungry and stop when satisfied.

5. **Balanced Meals:**
   - Ensure meals include a balance of protein, healthy fats, and fiber-rich carbohydrates for sustained energy.

6. **Plan Meals Ahead:**
   - Prepare meals and snacks in advance to avoid impulsive choices during eating windows.

7. Experiment with Timing:

- Explore different fasting windows to find what suits your schedule and lifestyle best.

8. Include Physical Activity:

- Incorporate regular exercise, but consider adjusting the intensity and timing based on your fasting schedule.

9. Stay Consistent:

- Aim for consistency in your eating and fasting times to help regulate your body's internal clock.

10. Manage Stress:

- Practice stress-reducing activities like meditation, deep breathing, or yoga to support overall well-being.

11. Seek Professional Guidance:

- Consult with a healthcare professional or nutritionist before starting intermittent fasting, especially if you have health concerns.

12. Be Patient:

- Allow time for your body to adapt to the new eating pattern, and be patient with the process.

13. Monitor Energy Levels:

- If you experience fatigue or other adverse effects, reassess your fasting strategy and make adjustments if needed.

14. **Social Considerations:**
   - Plan social events during eating windows to make fasting more manageable in social settings.

15. **Regular Check-Ins:**
   - Periodically evaluate how you feel physically and mentally to ensure that intermittent fasting aligns with your overall well-being.

Troubleshooting Common Challenges in Intermittent Fasting

1. **Overeating During Eating Windows**:
   - Focus on nutrient-dense foods to promote satiety.
   - Practice mindful eating, savoring each bite.

2. **Feeling Weak or Dizzy**:
   - Ensure you are staying hydrated, especially with water and electrolytes.
   - Consider adjusting fasting windows or meal composition.

3. **Difficulty Sleeping:**
   - Avoid large meals close to bedtime.

- Ensure you have enough time between your last meal and bedtime.

4. **Lack of Energy During Fasting:**
   - Choose nutrient-rich foods during eating windows.
   - Consider adjusting fasting times or patterns.

5. **Digestive Issues:**
   - Increase fiber intake gradually to allow your digestive system to adjust.
   - Stay hydrated to support healthy digestion.

6. **Social Challenges:**
   - Plan social activities during eating windows.
   - Communicate your fasting schedule with friends and family.

7. **Plateau in Weight Loss:**
   - Reevaluate your calorie intake and food choices.
   - Incorporate variations in your fasting routine.

8. **Hunger Pangs:**
   - Stay hydrated and drink water when hunger strikes.
   - Experiment with herbal teas or black coffee for appetite control.

9. **Feeling Irritable or Moody:**
   - Ensure you are meeting nutritional needs during eating windows.

  - Practice stress-management techniques.

10. **Cravings for Certain Foods:**
  - Allow occasional treats in moderation.
  - Find healthier alternatives to satisfy cravings.

11. **Inconsistent Results:**
  - Be patient and allow time for your body to adapt.
  - Adjust fasting strategies based on personal response.

12. **Medical Concerns:**
  - Consult with a healthcare professional if you have underlying health conditions or concerns about the impact of intermittent fasting on your health.

Physical Activity and Well-being during Intermittent Fasting

1. **Stay Active:**
  - Incorporate regular physical activity into your routine, including a mix of cardiovascular exercises, strength training, and flexibility exercises.

2. **Choose Convenient Times:**
  - Schedule workouts during periods when you're not fasting to ensure you have energy for exercise.

3. **Hydrate Before Exercise:**
   - Drink water before and after your workout to stay hydrated, especially if you're fasting.

4. **Consider Fasted Workouts:**
   - Some people prefer fasted workouts during their fasting period. Experiment and see what works best for your energy levels.

5. **Listen to Your Body:**
   - Pay attention to how your body responds to exercise during fasting. If you feel weak or dizzy, adjust your workout intensity or timing.

6. **Post-Workout Nutrition:**
   - After a workout, prioritize a balanced meal with protein, carbohydrates, and healthy fats to support recovery.

7. **Adapt to Your Routine:**
   - Adapt your exercise routine based on your fasting schedule and energy levels during eating windows.

8. **Include Rest Days:**
   - Allow for rest days to prevent burnout and support overall well-being.

9. **Mind-Body Activities:**

- Incorporate mind-body activities like yoga or meditation to manage stress and enhance overall well-being.

10. **Monitor Progress:**
   - Track your physical activity levels and well-being to assess the impact of intermittent fasting on your fitness goals.

11. **Stay Flexible:**
   - Be flexible with your exercise routine, adjusting it as needed to align with your fasting strategy and overall lifestyle.

12. **Prioritize Sleep:**
   - Ensure you're getting adequate sleep, as it plays a crucial role in recovery and overall well-being.

Incorporating Exercise into Your Intermittent Fasting Routine

1. **Schedule Regular Workouts:**
   - Plan consistent workout sessions during your eating windows for optimal energy levels.

2. **Mix Cardio and Strength Training:**

- Include a combination of cardiovascular exercises (e.g., walking, jogging) and strength training to promote overall fitness.

3. **Fasted Cardio, if Preferred:**
   - Some individuals prefer fasted cardio during their fasting period. Experiment to see if it suits your energy levels and preferences.

4. **High-Intensity Interval Training (HIIT):**
   - Incorporate HIIT workouts for efficient calorie burning and improved cardiovascular health.

5. **Enjoy Outdoor Activities:**
   - Engage in outdoor activities like hiking, cycling, or nature walks for a refreshing change.

6. **Prioritize Strength Training:**
   - Include strength training exercises to build muscle, enhance metabolism, and support overall body composition.

7. **Flexible Workout Times:**
   - Be flexible with your workout times, adjusting them based on your fasting schedule and daily routine.

8. **Post-Workout Nutrition:**
   - After workouts, consume a balanced meal with protein and carbohydrates to aid recovery.

9. **Rest and Recovery Days:**
   - Allow for rest and recovery days to prevent overtraining and support overall well-being.

10. **Mind-Body Activities:**
   - Incorporate activities like yoga or meditation to enhance flexibility, reduce stress, and promote mental well-being.

11. **Set Realistic Goals:**
   - Establish achievable fitness goals that align with your intermittent fasting plan and overall lifestyle.

12. **Stay Consistent:**
   - Consistency is key. Stick to your exercise routine and adjust as needed to accommodate fasting times.

13. **Hydrate Adequately:**
   - Drink water before, during, and after workouts to stay hydrated, especially if you're fasting.

14. **Track Progress:**
   - Monitor your fitness progress, whether it's improvements in strength, endurance, or overall well-being.

Mindful Practices for Holistic Health during Intermittent Fasting

1. **Mindful Eating:**
   - Pay attention to the flavors, textures, and sensations of each bite during your eating windows.
   - Chew your food slowly and savor each mouthful.

2. **Meditation:**
   - Incorporate mindfulness meditation to reduce stress and promote mental clarity.
   - Practice deep-breathing exercises during fasting periods.

3. **Yoga or Stretching:**
   - Engage in yoga or stretching exercises to enhance flexibility and promote relaxation.
   - Include gentle movements to align with your body's needs during fasting.

4. **Gratitude Journaling:**
   - Keep a gratitude journal to focus on positive aspects of your life, fostering a sense of contentment.

5. **Nature Walks:**
   - Take mindful walks in nature, appreciating the sights, sounds, and sensations around you.

6. Digital Detox:
   - Schedule periods of digital detox to reduce screen time and promote mental well-being.

7. Breathing Exercises:
   - Practice mindful breathing exercises to calm the mind and reduce stress levels.

8. Quality Sleep:
   - Prioritize a consistent sleep routine and create a calming bedtime environment for quality rest.

9. Body Scan Meditation:
   - Perform a body scan meditation to tune into sensations and release tension throughout the body.

10. Affirmations:
   - Incorporate positive affirmations to cultivate a positive mindset and boost self-confidence.

11. Hydration Awareness:
   - Be mindful of staying hydrated during fasting periods, sipping water mindfully.

12. Cultivate Joyful Activities:
   - Engage in activities that bring joy, whether it's reading, listening to music, or spending time with loved ones.

13. Mindful Work Breaks:
   - Take short breaks during work or daily activities to practice mindfulness, such as focusing on your breath or taking a mindful walk.

14. **Social Connection:**
   - Foster meaningful connections with others, whether through socializing or volunteering.

15. **Self-Compassion:**
   - Practice self-compassion and kindness toward yourself, especially during challenging moments.

Success Stories

1. **Weight Management:**
   - Many individuals report successful weight loss and improved body composition through intermittent fasting.

2. **Increased Energy:**
   - Some people note increased energy levels and improved focus during fasting periods.

3. **Simplified Eating Routine:**
   - Intermittent fasting can simplify meal planning and eliminate the need for frequent snacking.

4. **Enhanced Mental Clarity:**

- Improved mental clarity and concentration are often mentioned as positive outcomes.

5. Adaptability to Lifestyles:
- The flexibility of intermittent fasting allows people to adapt the eating pattern to their lifestyles.

6. Metabolic Benefits:
- Some studies suggest potential metabolic benefits, including improved insulin sensitivity and blood lipid profiles.

7. Lifestyle Sustainability:
- Individuals appreciate the sustainability of intermittent fasting as a long-term lifestyle choice.

8. Better Relationship with Food:
- Practicing mindful eating during eating windows can lead to a healthier relationship with food.

Conclusion

In conclusion, intermittent fasting is a lifestyle approach that has gained popularity for its potential health benefits. While success stories and positive outcomes are often reported, it's crucial to approach this eating pattern with careful consideration for individual health needs. Incorporating mindful practices, staying physically active, and making nutrient-dense food choices during eating windows can contribute to overall well-being.

Remember that there is no one-size-fits-all solution, and what works for one person may not work for another. If you're considering intermittent fasting, it's advisable to consult with healthcare professionals or nutritionists to ensure it aligns with your health goals and doesn't pose any risks, especially if you have underlying health conditions.

Ultimately, the key to success lies in finding a balanced approach that suits your lifestyle, supports your well-being, and aligns with your personal goals.

Final Thoughts and Encouragement

As you embark on your journey with intermittent fasting, keep in mind that it's a unique and personal experience. Embrace the process, listen to your body, and make adjustments that align with your well-being. Consistency, patience, and mindful practices can contribute to a positive and sustainable journey.

Remember, success is not solely measured by scale numbers or specific outcomes but by how well the lifestyle aligns with your overall health and happiness. Celebrate small victories, stay adaptable to your needs, and prioritize self-care throughout the process.

If challenges arise or if you have questions, seek guidance from healthcare professionals or nutrition experts who can provide personalized advice. Your health is a holistic journey, and intermittent fasting is just one aspect of it.

Wishing you a fulfilling and balanced experience as you explore the world of intermittent fasting. Here's to your health and well-being!